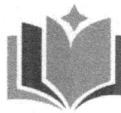

DB PUBLISHING

Top 10 Herbal Medicines for Everyday Life for Beginners

Table of Contents:

Introduction

Holistic medicine, also known as alternative or complementary medicine, is an approach to healthcare that considers the whole person—mind, body, and spirit—in the quest for optimal health and well-being. It emphasizes the integration of various modalities and addresses the underlying causes of illness rather than focusing on symptoms.

Having been around for thousands of years, holistic medicine acknowledges that the human body is a complex system with interconnected parts, and imbalances or disruptions in one area can affect the overall well-being. Therefore, it aims to promote harmony and balance within the individual by considering multiple factors such as lifestyle, nutrition, environment, emotions, and social interactions.

It's important to note that while holistic medicine can be beneficial for many individuals, it may not replace, but complement, conventional medical care. It is advisable to consult with qualified healthcare professionals and nutritionists to inform them about any holistic practices or therapies you may be considering.

What is Holistic Medicine?

1.	Individualized care: Holistic practitioners consider each person's unique circumstances and tailor treatments accordingly. They consider factors such as medical history, genetics, environment, and personal beliefs.

2.	Integration of modalities: Holistic medicine incorporates various healing approaches from both conventional medicine and alternative therapies (or natural medications that have been around for thousands of years). This may include conventional medical treatments, acupuncture, herbal medicine, nutritional counseling, mind-body techniques, energy healing, and more.

3.	Prevention and self-care: Holistic medicine emphasizes the importance of preventive measures and empowering individuals to take an active role in their own health. It encourages lifestyle changes, stress reduction techniques, healthy nutrition, exercise, and self-care practices.

4.	Mind-body connection: The interconnection between the mind, emotions, and physical health is recognized in holistic medicine. Techniques such as meditation, mindfulness, yoga, and psychotherapy may be employed to address emotional and psychological aspects of health.

5.	Emphasis on the root cause: Holistic medicine aims to identify and address the underlying causes of illness rather than merely suppressing symptoms. By treating the root cause, long-term healing and overall well-being can be achieved.

Benefits and Principles of Holistic Thinking

Holistic thinking is a comprehensive approach to improving all areas of life by considering the interconnectedness of mind, body, and spirit. It involves embracing alternative modalities such as herbal nutritionists, naturalists, and some chiropractors to gain a broader understanding of health and well-being. However, it is essential to maintain open communication with your primary physician and inform them of any lifestyle changes and reasons behind them.

Holistic thinking recognizes that optimal health goes beyond just physical well-being and encompasses emotional, mental, and spiritual aspects. By adopting this mindset, individuals can gain a more profound understanding of the root causes of imbalances and work towards achieving overall wellness.

Herbal nutritionists and naturalists can provide valuable insights into the healing power of herbs, plant-based remedies, and natural therapies. They can guide individuals in making informed decisions regarding nutrition, supplementation, and lifestyle adjustments that support their unique needs. Chiropractors, with their focus on spinal alignment and nervous system health, offer additional perspectives on holistic healing.

While incorporating holistic practices into your life, it is crucial to maintain a collaborative relationship with your primary physician. Informing them of your lifestyle changes and the reasons behind them helps ensure comprehensive care and enables them to assess the compatibility of various approaches with your specific health conditions and treatments.

Remember, holistic thinking is about integrating various modalities to enhance well-being, not replacing conventional medical care when necessary. By combining the insights of herbal nutritionists, naturalists, chiropractors, and your primary physician, you can cultivate a holistic approach that supports your overall health and fosters an empowered, balanced, and well-rounded life.

With that in mind, here are 10 commonly used holistic remedies, each of which will be discussed in more detail:

1.   Ginger: Known for its anti-inflammatory properties, ginger is often used to aid digestion, relieve nausea, and reduce muscle soreness.

2.   Turmeric: Curcumin, the active compound in turmeric, has potent anti-inflammatory and antioxidant effects, making it beneficial for conditions such as arthritis and digestive issues.

3.   Echinacea: Often used to support the immune system, echinacea is believed to help prevent and reduce the duration of colds and upper respiratory infections.

4.   Peppermint: Peppermint oil or tea can help alleviate symptoms of indigestion, including bloating, gas, and stomach discomfort.

5.   Chamomile: Chamomile tea is commonly used for its calming properties, helping to reduce anxiety, improve sleep quality, and soothe an upset stomach.

6.   Lavender: Lavender essential oil is often used in aromatherapy to promote relaxation and alleviate stress. It may also have mild pain-relieving properties.

7.   Valerian root: Valerian is a herb that is sometimes used as a natural sleep aid and is believed to help improve sleep quality and reduce insomnia symptoms.

8.   St. John's Wort: This herb has been used traditionally to manage symptoms of mild to moderate depression, although its use should be carefully monitored and discussed with a healthcare professional.

9.   Peppermint oil: Applied topically, peppermint oil can help relieve headaches, muscle tension, and provide a cooling sensation to the skin.

10.   Lemon balm: Often used as a calming herb, lemon balm may help reduce anxiety and promote relaxation.

These holistic remedies have been used for various conditions, but it's important to remember that individual results may vary. Always consult a nutritionist healthcare professional for advice tailored to your specific needs and health conditions.

Ginger: Nature's Digestive Healer

A Powerful Spice with Medicinal Properties and Digestive Health Benefits

Ginger, scientifically known as Zingiber Officinale, has been used for centuries not only as a culinary ingredient but also for its remarkable medicinal properties. This aromatic spice is not only known for adding a delightful kick to dishes but also for its potential health benefits, particularly in promoting digestive health. In this informational guide, we will explore the medicinal properties and digestive health benefits of ginger.

Medicinal Properties of Ginger:

1.   Anti-inflammatory properties: Ginger contains bioactive compounds such as gingerols and shogaols, which possess potent anti-inflammatory effects. These compounds help reduce inflammation in the body, making ginger beneficial for individuals suffering from conditions like arthritis and inflammatory bowel disease.

2.   Anti-nausea and anti-vomiting effects: Ginger has long been used to alleviate nausea and vomiting caused by motion sickness, morning sickness during pregnancy, and chemotherapy-induced nausea. It acts on the digestive system, helping to calm an upset stomach and prevent vomiting.

Digestive Health Benefits of Ginger:

1.   Relieves indigestion: Ginger stimulates the production of digestive enzymes, aiding in the breakdown of food and improving digestion. It can alleviate symptoms of indigestion, including bloating, flatulence, and discomfort after meals.

2.   Reduces gastrointestinal spasms: Ginger's antispasmodic properties help relax the muscles of the gastrointestinal tract, relieving cramps and spasms. This can be particularly beneficial for individuals with irritable bowel syndrome (IBS).

3.   Enhances nutrient absorption: By improving digestion, ginger promotes better nutrient absorption in the intestines. This ensures that the body can effectively utilize the essential vitamins, minerals, and other nutrients from the food we consume.

4.   Anti-microbial effects: Ginger exhibits antimicrobial activity against various pathogens, including bacteria like E. coli and H. pylori. This can help prevent infections and support a healthy balance of gut bacteria.

Incorporating Ginger into Your Diet: To harness the medicinal and digestive health benefits of ginger, you can incorporate it into your diet in various ways:

1.   Fresh ginger: Add grated or sliced ginger to your teas, soups, stir-fries, and salad dressings.

2.   Ginger tea: Steep fresh ginger slices in hot water for a soothing and invigorating beverage.

3.   Ginger supplements: If incorporating ginger into your diet is challenging, consider ginger supplements available in capsule or powder form. However, consult your healthcare provider before starting any new supplements.

Ginger is a versatile spice with a wide range of medicinal properties and digestive health benefits. Its anti-inflammatory, anti-nausea, and digestive-enhancing effects make it a valuable addition to a healthy lifestyle. By including ginger in your diet, you can potentially experience relief from digestive discomfort and support your overall well-being. Remember to consult a healthcare professional if you have any specific health concerns or if you are considering ginger as a supplement.

Turmeric:

The Golden Spice of Healing

Nature's Anti-Inflammatory Powerhouse

Turmeric, derived from the plant Curcuma longa, is a vibrant golden spice commonly used in Indian cuisine. Beyond its culinary uses, turmeric has gained popularity for its impressive anti-inflammatory properties. In this informational guide, we will explore the potential health benefits of turmeric and its role in reducing inflammation in the body.

Understanding Turmeric's Anti-Inflammatory Properties:

1.   Curcumin, the active compound: The key component responsible for turmeric's anti-inflammatory effects is curcumin. Curcumin is a powerful antioxidant and exhibits strong anti-inflammatory properties, making turmeric a valuable natural remedy.

2.   Inhibition of inflammatory molecules: Curcumin inhibits various molecules and enzymes involved in the inflammatory response, including cytokines, COX-2, and NF-κB. By modulating these inflammatory pathways, turmeric can help reduce chronic inflammation in the body.

3.   Reduction of oxidative stress: Oxidative stress plays a significant role in inflammation and various chronic diseases. Curcumin's antioxidant properties neutralize free radicals and reduce oxidative stress, contributing to its anti-inflammatory effects.

Potential Health Benefits of Turmeric's Anti-Inflammatory Properties:

1.   Alleviation of joint pain and arthritis: Turmeric's anti-inflammatory properties may help alleviate joint pain and stiffness associated with conditions like osteoarthritis and rheumatoid arthritis. It can potentially reduce swelling, improve mobility, and enhance overall joint health.

2.   Support for digestive health: Turmeric stimulates the production of bile, aiding digestion and supporting liver function. It may alleviate symptoms of inflammatory bowel disease (IBD) and promote a healthy digestive system.

3.   Cardiovascular health: Chronic inflammation is linked to cardiovascular diseases. Turmeric's anti-inflammatory properties, along with its potential to improve cholesterol levels and prevent blood clot formation, may contribute to a healthier heart.

4.   Brain health and cognitive function: Inflammation is associated with neurodegenerative diseases like Alzheimer's and Parkinson's. Turmeric's anti-inflammatory effects, coupled with its antioxidant properties, may help protect brain cells, improve memory, and support cognitive function.

Incorporating Turmeric into Your Diet: To reap the anti-inflammatory benefits of turmeric, consider these tips:

1.   Golden milk: Prepare a comforting drink by combining turmeric, warm milk (dairy or plant-based), a pinch of black pepper (which enhances curcumin absorption), and a natural sweetener like honey.

2.   Turmeric in cooking: Add turmeric powder to your curries, soups, stews, and roasted vegetables to infuse them with its vibrant color and health benefits.

3.   Turmeric supplements: If incorporating turmeric into your diet is challenging, consider turmeric supplements standardized for curcumin content.

Turmeric, with its active compound curcumin, offers potent anti-inflammatory properties that can have a positive impact on overall health and well-being. By incorporating turmeric into your diet or considering curcumin supplements, you may experience reduced inflammation, relief from joint pain, improved digestive health, and potential benefits for cardiovascular and brain health. Embrace the golden spice and harness nature's anti-inflammatory powerhouse for a healthier lifestyle. Remember to consult a healthcare professional/nutritionist for personalized advice, especially if you have underlying health conditions.

Echinacea:

Boosting Immunity Naturally

Boosting Immunity and Guarding Against Colds and Flu

Echinacea, a flowering plant native to North America, has a long history of traditional use for its immune-boosting properties. In this informational guide, we will explore the potential health benefits of echinacea, its role in strengthening the immune system, and its effectiveness in preventing and preparing for colds and flu.

Strengthening the Immune System:

1.   Immune-enhancing compounds: Echinacea contains bioactive compounds, including flavonoids, polysaccharides, and alkamides, which can stimulate the immune system. These compounds activate immune cells, enhance their activity, and promote the production of cytokines, proteins that regulate immune responses.

2.   Anti-inflammatory effects: Echinacea possesses anti-inflammatory properties that help reduce inflammation in the body. By modulating inflammatory responses, echinacea supports overall immune function and helps combat various infections.

Cold and Flu Prevention:

1.   Reducing the severity and duration of symptoms: Echinacea may help reduce the severity and duration of cold and flu symptoms. Studies suggest that regular echinacea use at the onset of symptoms can alleviate symptoms such as sore throat, congestion, and coughing.

2.   Antiviral activity: Echinacea exhibits antiviral properties and can help inhibit the replication of viruses, including those that cause colds and flu. By preventing the proliferation of viral particles, echinacea may assist in preventing the onset or progression of these infections.

Preparing Echinacea Preparations:

1.   Echinacea supplements: Echinacea is available in various forms, including capsules, tablets, liquid extracts, and tinctures. When choosing a supplement, look for standardized extracts with a high content of echinacea's active compounds. Follow the recommended dosage instructions and consult a healthcare professional if you have specific health concerns or are taking other medications.

2.   Echinacea tea: You can prepare echinacea tea by steeping dried echinacea root or leaves in hot water for 10-15 minutes. Strain the tea and enjoy it up to three times a day. Note that echinacea tea may have a bitter taste, so you can add honey or lemon to enhance the flavor.

3.   Topical applications: Echinacea creams or ointments can be used topically to soothe skin irritations, cuts, or minor wounds. Apply them directly to the affected area as needed, following the product instructions.

Echinacea offers promising immune-boosting properties and has been traditionally used to prevent and manage colds and flu. By incorporating echinacea supplements or preparing echinacea tea, you can potentially strengthen your immune system, reduce the severity of symptoms, and aid in cold and flu prevention. Remember to consult a healthcare professional before starting any new supplements, especially if you have underlying health conditions or are taking other medications. Embrace the power of echinacea to support your immune health and maintain well-being during cold and flu seasons.

Peppermint:

A Fresh Approach to Wellness

A Refreshing Herb with Digestive, Headache, and Muscle Pain Benefits

Peppermint, known scientifically as Mentha × Piperita, is a popular herb known for its refreshing aroma and numerous health benefits. In this informational guide, we will explore the potential effects of peppermint on digestion, headaches, muscle pain, and its versatile potential in various applications.

Improving Digestion:

1.   Relieving digestive discomfort: Peppermint has been used for centuries to alleviate symptoms such as bloating, indigestion, and stomach cramps. Its active compound, menthol, relaxes the smooth muscles in the gastrointestinal tract, promoting smoother digestion and relieving spasms.

2.   Managing irritable bowel syndrome (IBS): Peppermint oil has shown promising results in managing symptoms of IBS, including abdominal pain, bloating, and changes in bowel patterns. It may help reduce the severity and frequency of IBS episodes, improving overall quality of life.

Headache Relief:

1.   Cooling and analgesic effects: Peppermint's cooling properties provide a soothing sensation that can help relieve tension headaches. Applying peppermint oil (later in book) to the temples or forehead may provide a refreshing, cooling effect and potentially reduce headache pain.

2.   Promoting relaxation: Peppermint's aroma has been associated with stress reduction and relaxation. Inhaling peppermint essential oil or using it in aromatherapy may help alleviate headache symptoms induced by stress or tension.

Muscle Pain Relief:

1.   Muscle relaxant properties: Peppermint oil, when applied topically, has a cooling and numbing effect on muscles. It can help alleviate muscle pain, soreness, and tension. Consider using peppermint-infused balms, creams, or massage oils to target specific areas of discomfort.

2.   Reducing exercise-induced muscle soreness: Peppermint oil, with its potential anti-inflammatory properties, may help reduce inflammation and muscle soreness following intense physical activity. Mixing a few drops of peppermint oil with a carrier oil and massaging it into the affected muscles may aid in recovery.

Potential Applications and Precautions:

1.   Culinary uses: Peppermint leaves can be used in various culinary creations, including teas, beverages, desserts, and savory dishes. It adds a refreshing flavor and aroma to recipes.

2.   Essential oil caution: While peppermint essential oil offers many benefits, it is highly concentrated and should be used with caution. Always dilute it in a carrier oil before applying topically. Consult a healthcare professional for proper guidance, especially if you have sensitive skin or are pregnant.

Peppermint is a versatile herb known for its beneficial effects on digestion, headaches, and muscle pain. Whether enjoyed as a tea, used topically in essential oil form, or incorporated into culinary delights, peppermint offers a refreshing and natural approach to promote well-being. However, it's important to exercise caution and consult a healthcare professional for personalized advice, especially if you have specific health conditions or concerns. Embrace the invigorating properties of peppermint to enhance your digestive health, find headache relief, and soothe muscle discomfort.

Chamomile:

Tranquility in a Teacup

Calming the Nervous System, Promoting Sleep, and Beautifying Skin

Chamomile, derived from the daisy-like flowers of the Matricaria Chamomilla plant, has been valued for centuries for its soothing and therapeutic properties. In this informational guide, we will explore the influence of chamomile on the nervous system, its ability to promote restful sleep, and its applications in beauty and skincare.

Influence on the Nervous System:

1.   Calming effects: Chamomile is known for its calming and relaxing properties. It contains compounds such as apigenin and bisabolol that interact with receptors in the brain, promoting feelings of relaxation and reducing anxiety.

2.   Stress management: Chamomile's calming effects make it beneficial for managing stress and tension. Consuming chamomile tea or using chamomile in aromatherapy can help alleviate symptoms of stress, promoting a sense of well-being.

Promoting Restful Sleep:

1.   Sleep aid: Chamomile is renowned for its sleep-inducing properties. Drinking chamomile tea before bedtime can help improve sleep quality, reduce insomnia, and ease restlessness. Its mild sedative effects may be attributed to the compound apigenin, which binds to certain receptors in the brain associated with sleep.

2.   Relaxing bedtime routine: Incorporating chamomile into your bedtime routine can signal to your body that it's time to unwind and prepare for sleep. Enjoying a warm cup of chamomile tea or using chamomile-infused pillow sprays or bath products can create a calming environment conducive to a good night's rest.

Beauty and Skincare Applications:

1.   Skin-soothing properties: Chamomile's anti-inflammatory and antioxidant properties make it a valuable ingredient in skincare. It can help calm and soothe irritated skin, reduce redness, and promote a healthy complexion.

2.   Gentle cleansing: Chamomile is often used in facial cleansers or toners due to its mild astringent properties. It can help cleanse and purify the skin without causing excessive dryness or irritation.

3.   Enhancing hair color and shine: Chamomile is known for its ability to enhance golden tones in blonde or light brown hair. Rinsing hair with chamomile-infused water or using chamomile-based hair products can add natural highlights and impart a healthy shine.

Chamomile's influence on the nervous system, sleep promotion, and beauty and skincare applications make it a versatile and beneficial herb. Whether sipping a warm cup of chamomile tea to unwind, incorporating chamomile-infused skincare products into your routine, or using chamomile for its hair-enhancing properties, chamomile offers natural and soothing benefits. However, it's important to note that individual responses may vary, and if you have specific health concerns or allergies, it is advisable to consult with a healthcare professional. Embrace the calming and beautifying powers of chamomile to nurture your overall well-being, achieve a restful sleep, and enhance your natural beauty.

Lavender:

A Fragrant Oasis of Serenity

Nature's Soothing Essence for Stress Reduction, Anxiety, Skin Care, and First Aid

Lavender, with its delicate purple flowers and enchanting aroma, is more than just a beautiful plant. It has been revered for its versatile therapeutic properties. From its calming effects on the mind and body to its remarkable benefits for skin care and first aid, lavender offers a holistic approach to wellness. Let's explore its remarkable abilities.

Stress Reduction and Anxiety Relief: Lavender's soothing scent has been widely used in aromatherapy to promote relaxation and reduce stress. Inhaling lavender essential oil can help calm the nervous system, ease tension, and induce a sense of tranquility. It has shown promising results in reducing anxiety symptoms and improving sleep quality. Whether through diffusers, sachets, or diluted oil applied to pulse points, lavender can provide a much-needed respite from the demands of everyday life.

Skin Care and First Aid: Lavender possesses antiseptic and anti-inflammatory properties, making it a valuable addition to any skincare routine. It can help soothe irritated skin, reduce redness, and promote wound healing. Lavender oil can be added to carrier oils or creams to create a gentle and effective skincare product. It is also known to relieve discomfort caused by insect bites, minor burns, and cuts. Diluted lavender oil applied topically can help alleviate pain and accelerate the healing process.

Usage Tips: To benefit from the effects of lavender, consider the following tips:

• Aromatherapy: Add a few drops of lavender essential oil to a diffuser or inhale directly from the bottle for a calming effect.

• Bathing: Add a few drops of lavender oil to your bathwater for a relaxing soak.

• Massage: Blend lavender oil with a carrier oil (such as almond or coconut oil) for a soothing massage experience.

• Skincare: Mix a few drops of lavender oil with your preferred carrier oil or lotion for gentle skincare.

• First Aid: Dilute lavender oil in a carrier oil and apply it to minor cuts, burns, or insect bites.

Remember to perform a patch test before using lavender oil topically and consult with a healthcare professional if you have any specific concerns or medical conditions.

Incorporating lavender into your daily life can help create a calming sanctuary amidst the chaos. So, take a deep breath, let the aroma of lavender envelop your senses, and embrace the gentle healing it offers for stress reduction, anxiety relief, skincare, and first aid.

Valerian Root:

Unleashing the Power of Restful Sleep

A Natural Remedy for Insomnia and Nervous System Support

Valerian root, derived from the Valeriana Officinalis plant, has been used for centuries as a natural remedy for sleep issues and nervous system support. In this informational guide, we will explore the effects of valerian root on insomnia, its influence on the nervous system, and its usage considerations and potential side effects.

Insomnia Relief:

1.   Sleep-promoting properties: Valerian root is renowned for its ability to promote relaxation and improve sleep quality. Its compounds, such as Valerenic Acid, interact with gamma-aminobutyric acid (GABA) receptors in the brain, leading to a calming effect and aiding in sleep initiation.

2.   Insomnia management: Valerian root can be effective in managing mild to moderate insomnia. It may help reduce the time required to fall asleep, increase total sleep time, and improve sleep quality.

Support for the Nervous System:

1.   Anxiety reduction: Valerian root has anxiolytic properties that can help alleviate symptoms of anxiety and nervousness. By enhancing the effects of GABA, valerian root promotes a sense of calmness and relaxation.

2.   Stress management: Valerian root may assist in managing stress-related symptoms. Its soothing properties can

help reduce feelings of restlessness and tension, contributing to an overall sense of well-being.

Usage and Potential Side Effects:

1.   Dosage and forms: Valerian root is available in various forms, including capsules, tablets, liquid extracts, and teas. Follow the instructions on the product label or consult a healthcare professional for appropriate dosing recommendations.

2.   Timing considerations: Valerian root is best taken approximately one hour before bedtime to facilitate sleep. Allow enough time for the effects to kick in before retiring for the night.

3.   Potential side effects: While generally considered safe, valerian root may cause mild side effects in some individuals. These may include drowsiness, dizziness, headache, stomach upset, or vivid dreams. It is recommended to start with a low dose to gauge individual tolerance.

4.   Interactions and precautions: Valerian root may interact with certain medications, such as sedatives, anti-anxiety drugs, or antihistamines. Consult with a healthcare professional if you have underlying health conditions, are taking medications, or are pregnant or breastfeeding.

Valerian root offers a natural approach to insomnia relief and nervous system support. Its sleep-promoting and calming effects can aid in managing sleep issues and promoting relaxation. While generally well-tolerated, it is important to be aware of potential side effects and consult with a healthcare professional before use. Embrace the soothing benefits of valerian root as a natural remedy to enhance sleep quality and support a calm and balanced nervous system.

St. John's Wort:

Finding Light in the Shadows

Enhancing Mood and Emotional Well-Being, Exploring its Role in Depression, and Important Precautions

St. John's Wort, scientifically known as Hypericum Perforatum, is a medicinal herb renowned for its potential mood-enhancing properties. In this informational guide, we will delve into the effects of St. John's Wort on mood enhancement, emotional well-being, its role in depression management, and important precautions to consider.

Mood Enhancement and Emotional Well-Being:

1.   Serotonin modulation: St. John's Wort is believed to increase the availability of serotonin in the brain, a neurotransmitter associated with mood regulation. By modulating serotonin levels, it may contribute to an overall improvement in mood and emotional well-being.

2.   Stress reduction: St. John's Wort has adaptogenic properties, helping the body adapt to stress and potentially reducing feelings of anxiety and tension. It may assist in managing mild to moderate symptoms of stress-related conditions.

Managing Depression:

1.   Mild to moderate depression: St. John's Wort has been studied for its potential in managing mild to moderate depression. Some studies suggest that it may be as effective as certain conventional antidepressant medications. However, it is

crucial to consult a healthcare professional for a proper diagnosis and guidance.

2.   Serotonin regulation: Similar to its mood-enhancing effects, St. John's Wort's ability to modulate serotonin levels may contribute to its potential benefits in depression management. It may help alleviate depressive symptoms such as sadness, lack of energy, and changes in appetite.

Important Precautions:

1.   Consultation with healthcare professionals: Before using St. John's Wort, it is essential to consult with a healthcare professional, especially if you have a history of depression or are taking medications. St. John's Wort may interact with various medications, including antidepressants, birth control pills, and blood thinners.

2.   Photosensitivity: St. John's Wort may cause increased sensitivity to sunlight, resulting in a higher risk of sunburn or skin irritation. If using St. John's Wort, minimize sun exposure and use appropriate sun protection.

3.   Side effects and dosage: St. John's Wort may cause side effects such as gastrointestinal upset, dizziness, or dry mouth. Adhere to the recommended dosage and be vigilant for any adverse reactions. Discontinue use and consult a healthcare professional if any unusual symptoms arise.

St. John's Wort offers potential mood-enhancing benefits and may contribute to emotional well-being. While it has been studied for its role in managing mild to moderate depression, it is crucial to seek professional advice for a proper diagnosis and treatment plan. Adherence to precautions, such as consulting with healthcare professionals and being mindful of potential interactions and photosensitivity, is essential. Explore the potential benefits of St. John's Wort as a natural approach to mood enhancement and emotional support, but always prioritize personalized healthcare guidance for optimal well-being.

Peppermint Oil:

Essential for Holistic Health

A Natural Solution for Pain Relief and Headache Management, and Proper Usage Techniques

Peppermint oil is an essential oil extracted from the leaves of the peppermint plant. It is obtained through a process of steam distillation or cold-pressing. Peppermint oil contains concentrated amounts of the beneficial compounds found in the peppermint plant, including menthol, menthone, and menthyl acetate. These compounds give peppermint oil its characteristic aroma, taste, and therapeutic properties. Peppermint oil is highly potent and is typically used in small amounts for its medicinal, aromatic, or topical benefits.

Pain Relief:

1.   Cooling and analgesic effects: Peppermint oil possesses a cooling sensation when applied topically, which can provide temporary pain relief. Its analgesic properties help alleviate muscle and joint discomfort, headaches, and minor injuries.

2.   Muscle relaxation: Peppermint oil's muscle-relaxing properties make it effective for soothing tension and easing muscle cramps. Applying diluted peppermint oil to the affected area can help reduce pain and promote relaxation.

Headache Management:

1.   Soothing tension headaches: Peppermint oil is commonly used to manage tension headaches due to its cooling and analgesic effects. Dilute a few drops of peppermint

oil in a carrier oil and apply it to the temples and forehead for relief.

2.   Reducing migraine symptoms: Peppermint oil has shown promise in reducing the intensity and duration of migraines. It can be applied topically or inhaled for its calming effects during a migraine attack.

Proper Usage Techniques:

1.   Topical application: To use peppermint oil topically, always dilute it with a suitable carrier oil like coconut or jojoba oil. The recommended dilution ratio is typically 2-3 drops of peppermint oil per teaspoon of carrier oil. Apply the mixture to the desired area and massage gently.

2.   Inhalation: Inhalation of peppermint oil can provide relief for headaches and sinus congestion. Add a few drops of peppermint oil to a diffuser, inhale it directly from the bottle, or dilute it in hot water for steam inhalation.

3.   Patch test: Before using peppermint oil topically, perform a patch test on a small area of skin to check for any adverse reactions or sensitivities. If redness, itching, or irritation occurs, discontinue use.

4.   Avoid contact with sensitive areas: Peppermint oil can be irritating to sensitive areas such as the eyes and mucous membranes. Use caution and avoid direct contact with these areas. If accidental contact occurs, rinse thoroughly with cool water.

Peppermint oil offers a natural and versatile solution for pain relief, particularly for headaches and muscle discomfort. When used properly, it can provide a cooling and soothing effect to ease tension and promote relaxation. Remember to dilute peppermint oil before topical use and perform a patch test to ensure compatibility with your skin. Whether applied topically or inhaled, peppermint oil can be an effective addition to your holistic wellness routine. If you have specific health concerns or are pregnant or breastfeeding, consult a healthcare professional before using peppermint oil. Embrace the natural benefits of peppermint oil for pain relief and headache management and enjoy the refreshing aroma it brings to your well-being.

Lemon Balm:

A Zest for Peace and Balance

An Herbal Remedy for Anxiety, Relaxation, Cognitive Support, and Creative Uses in Daily Life

Lemon balm, scientifically known as Melissa Officinalis, is a fragrant herb with a long history of use for its calming and therapeutic properties. In this informational guide, we will explore the effects of lemon balm on anxiety reduction, relaxation, cognitive support, and creative ways to incorporate it into daily life.

Anxiety Reduction and Relaxation:

1.	Calming properties: Lemon balm has been traditionally used to alleviate anxiety and promote relaxation. It contains compounds, including Rosmarinus Acid and flavonoids, which may help reduce stress and enhance feelings of calmness.

2.	Mood regulation: Lemon balm may assist in stabilizing mood by modulating neurotransmitters such as GABA (gamma-aminobutyric acid). Increasing GABA activity can induce relaxation and a sense of well-being.

Cognitive Support:

1.	Memory and concentration: Lemon balm may have positive effects on cognitive function, including memory and concentration. Studies suggest that it may improve cognitive performance and contribute to mental clarity and focus.

2.	Stress-related cognitive decline: Chronic stress can impact cognitive function, and lemon balm's stress-reducing properties may help protect against stress-related cognitive decline. By alleviating stress, lemon balm may support overall cognitive health.

Creative Uses in Daily Life:

1.   Herbal tea: Enjoy lemon balm as a soothing herbal tea by steeping fresh or dried lemon balm leaves in hot water. Sip it throughout the day to promote relaxation and clarity of mind.

2.   Aromatherapy: Inhale the calming scent of lemon balm essential oil through a diffuser or by adding a few drops to a warm bath. This can help create a peaceful and rejuvenating atmosphere.

3.   Culinary delights: Add fresh lemon balm leaves to salads, smoothies, or infused water for a refreshing and aromatic twist. It can also be used to garnish desserts or as a flavoring agent in various culinary creations.

4.   DIY skincare: Create homemade skincare products by infusing lemon balm leaves into oils or using them in facial steams. Lemon balm's antioxidant properties can help soothe and nourish the skin.

Lemon balm offers a range of benefits, including anxiety reduction, relaxation, cognitive support, and creative applications in daily life. Whether sipping a cup of lemon balm tea, enjoying the calming aroma through aromatherapy, or incorporating it into culinary and skincare endeavors, lemon balm can enhance well-being and inspire creativity. Embrace this versatile herb to promote relaxation, support cognitive function, and infuse your daily life with its refreshing qualities. Remember to consult a healthcare professional if you have specific health concerns or are taking medications. Discover the natural benefits of lemon balm and let its soothing effects and creative potential enrich your daily routine.

Holistic Health: A Personal Journey

Finding Balance in Mind, Body, and Spirit:

Incorporating Holistic Medications into Daily Routines for Lifestyle Changes

Achieving balance in mind, body, and spirit is essential for overall well-being and a harmonious life. One way to cultivate this balance is by incorporating holistic medications into daily routines. In this informational guide, we will explore the integration of holistic medications into daily life, fostering lifestyle changes that promote balance and enhance holistic well-being.

1.   Mind: a) Meditation and mindfulness: Practice meditation or mindfulness techniques daily to calm the mind, improve focus, and cultivate inner peace. Set aside dedicated time for quiet reflection and self-awareness.

b) Cognitive exercises: Engage in activities that stimulate the mind, such as reading, solving puzzles, or learning new skills. These exercises enhance mental agility, promote creativity, and support overall cognitive health.

2.   Body: a) Physical activity: Engage in regular exercise that suits your preferences and abilities. Whether it's yoga, walking, dancing, or strength training, physical activity boosts energy levels, improves mood, and supports physical health.

b) Holistic nutrition: Make conscious food choices that nourish your body. Focus on incorporating whole foods, fruits, vegetables, lean proteins, and healthy fats into your diet. Stay hydrated and avoid processed foods and excessive sugar and caffeine intake.

3.   Spirit: a) Spiritual practices: Explore spiritual practices that resonate with you, such as prayer, gratitude exercises, journaling or connecting with nature. These practices foster a sense of connection, purpose, and inner harmony.

b) Holistic therapies: Consider holistic therapies like acupuncture, Reiki, Healing Touch therapy or aromatherapy to align and balance your energy centers. These therapies can enhance spiritual well-being and promote a sense of holistic harmony.

4.   Integrating Holistic Medications: a) Herbal remedies: Incorporate herbal remedies such as chamomile tea, lavender oil, or ashwagandha supplements into your daily routine to support relaxation, stress reduction, and overall well-being.

b) Essential oils: Utilize essential oils like peppermint, eucalyptus, or frankincense in aromatherapy or as natural remedies for specific needs, such as calming the mind, uplifting the mood, or promoting sleep.

c) Holistic supplements: Consult with a healthcare professional to identify holistic supplements that support your specific needs, such as omega-3 fatty acids for brain health or probiotics for gut health.

Conclusion: By integrating holistic medications into daily routines and embracing lifestyle changes, you can nurture balance in mind, body, and spirit. Through practices like meditation, physical activity, mindful nutrition, and spiritual exploration, you create a foundation for holistic well-being. Additionally, incorporating herbal remedies, essential oils, and holistic supplements further enhances your journey towards balance. Remember to approach these practices with openness, adapt them to your individual needs, and consult healthcare professionals when necessary. Embrace the transformative power of holistic medications and lifestyle changes and discover a more balanced and vibrant life in mind, body, and spirit.

Embracing Power of Holistic Healing

Embracing holistic healing can lead to potential cost savings on doctor visits, prescription medications, and insurance. By focusing on preventive care, incorporating natural remedies, and adopting a healthy lifestyle, you can reduce the need for frequent doctor visits and costly treatments. Holistic practices such as proper nutrition, exercise, meditation, and stress reduction can promote overall well-being, minimizing the reliance on prescription drugs. While it's important to consult healthcare professionals for serious conditions, embracing holistic healing can empower you to take charge of your health, potentially saving money in the long run and leading to a more balanced and sustainable approach to wellness.

A Surprise! ALOE!!!!!

Cutting, Eating, and Digestive Benefits with Delicious Recipes

Aloe vera, a succulent plant with gel-filled leaves, is renowned for its medicinal properties and digestive benefits. In this informational guide, we will explore the process of cutting and eating aloe vera, as well as its effects on the digestive system. Additionally, we will provide delicious recipes that incorporate aloe vera for a wholesome culinary experience.

Cutting and Eating Aloe Vera:

> *Harvesting the gel*: Select mature aloe vera leaves and carefully cut them close to the base. Rinse the leaves to remove any dirt or residue. To extract the gel, (options) 1 - slice through the leaf lengthwise and use a spoon to scoop out the clear gel. 2 – use a potato peeler to remove the spines, green shell, and base of the leaf.

> *Preparing the gel*: Rinse (place in cup of water for a few minutes, then quick rinse) the gel to remove the yellow latex, which can have a bitter taste and potential laxative effect. Once cleaned, dice or blend the gel into a smooth consistency suitable for consumption. OR, just put it in water and let it liquify. The water will become very thick but drinkable (esp for those who aspirate easily, this is best). Drink a cup and add water back into the original gel and let the liquification continue until the water is near its normal consistency, then just eat the gel!! It's nearly tasteless!

Digestive Benefits:

1.   Soothing properties: Aloe vera gel contains compounds like polysaccharides that possess soothing and anti-inflammatory effects. When consumed, it can help soothe the digestive tract, alleviating conditions such as acid reflux, heartburn, and irritable bowel syndrome (IBS).

2.   Promoting gut health: Aloe vera has prebiotic properties that support the growth of beneficial gut bacteria. This can contribute to a healthy gut microbiome, which is essential for proper digestion and overall well-being.

Delicious Aloe Vera Recipes:

1.   Aloe Vera Smoothie:

•   Blend 2-3 tablespoons of aloe vera gel, 1 cup of coconut water, 1 ripe banana, a handful of spinach, and a squeeze of fresh lemon juice. Enjoy a refreshing and nutrient-packed smoothie to kickstart your day.

2.   Aloe Vera Salad Dressing:

•   Mix 2 tablespoons of aloe vera gel, 1 tablespoon of extra virgin olive oil, 1 tablespoon of apple cider vinegar, a pinch of salt, and a dash of honey. Drizzle this flavorful dressing over your favorite salad for a healthy twist.

3.   Aloe Vera Yogurt Parfait:

•   Layer Greek yogurt, diced aloe vera gel, fresh berries, and a sprinkle of granola or nuts in a glass. This colorful and nourishing parfait makes for a delightful breakfast or healthy dessert option.

Note: It is important to exercise caution when consuming aloe vera, as some individuals may experience adverse reactions or allergies. Start with small amounts to gauge your body's response and consult a healthcare professional if you have any concerns or specific health conditions.

Incorporating aloe vera into your diet can offer numerous digestive benefits. By cutting and properly preparing the gel, you can create delicious recipes that provide soothing properties and support gut health. Embrace the versatility of aloe vera as an ingredient in smoothies, salad dressings, parfaits, or drink it liquified while reaping its digestive rewards. As with any dietary changes, listen to your body and consult a healthcare nutritionist professional if needed. Enjoy the nourishing and refreshing effects of aloe vera as you embark on a journey toward better digestive health.

We hope you enjoyed the book. Please leave a review and let us know what you think.

Author's Page

Love this book?

**CHECK OUT MORE
BY SCANNING
THIS QR CODE.**

SCAN ME

9 789898 956095